Intermittent Fasting

A Guide to a Healthy Life

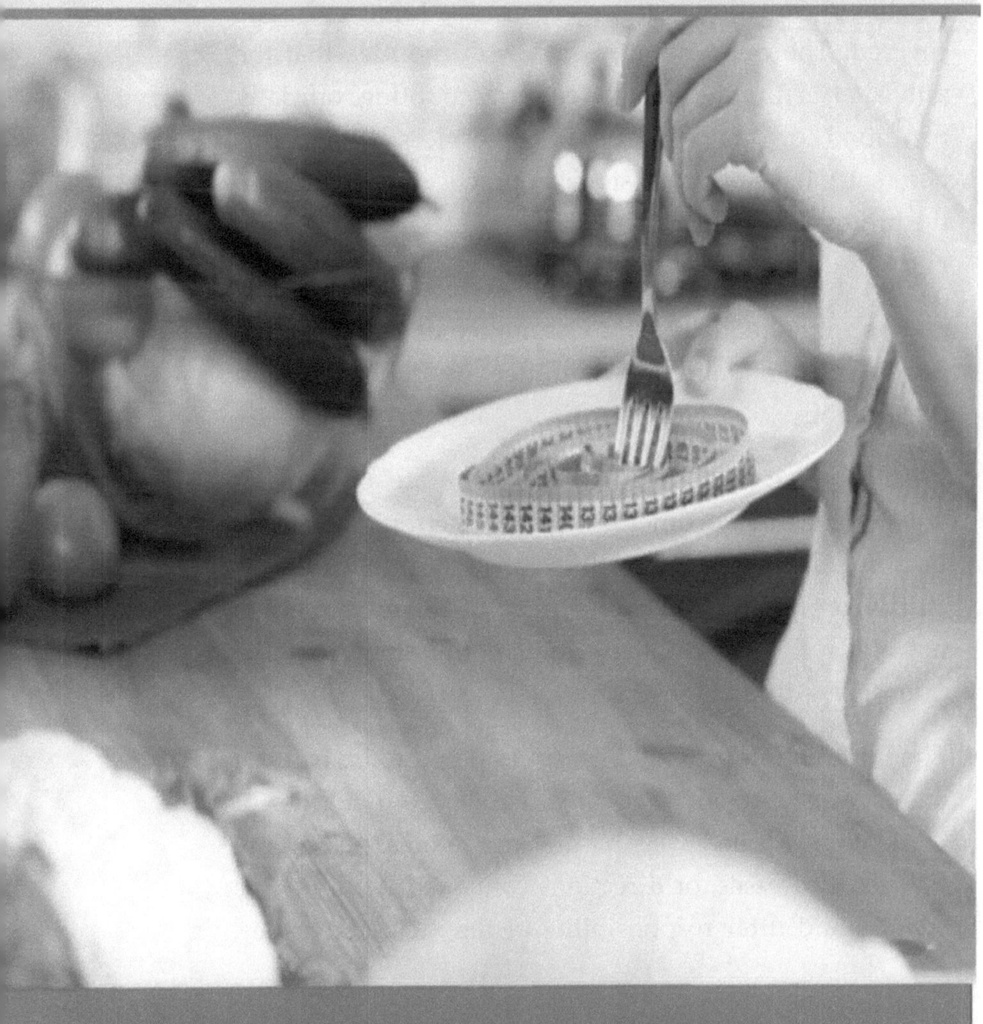

Terry Dunlap

Disclaimer

All erudition contained in this book is given for informational and educational purposes only. The author is not in any way accountable for any results or outcomes that emanate from using this material. Constructive attempts have been made to provide information that is both accurate and effective, but the author is not bound for the accuracy or use/misuse of this information.

Contents

FOREWORD

First, I will like to thank you for taking the first step of trusting me and deciding to purchase/read this life-transforming eBook. Thanks for spending your time and resources on this material.

I can assure you of exact results if you will diligently follow the exact blueprint, I lay bare in the information manual you are currently reading. It has transformed lives, and I strongly believe it will equally transform your own life too.

All the information I presented in this Do It Yourself piece is easy to digest and practice.

INTRODUCTION

Hello my name is Terry Dunlap and I have successfully lost 55 pounds in 10 weeks by intermittent fasting. I noticed that my clothes where getting tighter and I was really packing on the weight. I work a full-time job and I also have 3 kids to look after. So, I had very little time for exercising at a gym. So, I looked for ways I could lose the weight without having to go to the gym and I came across some articles on intermittent fasting. I am the type of guy who wants the fastest result in as little time as possible. I did the 20:4 method and eating healthy instantly. A week into fasting I lost 7 pounds. My mind was blown and I couldn't believe the results. The following week I lost 6 pounds. About a month into fasting I decided to kick it up another level by exercising and I could see my body transform.

So, after trying this out and with the way it worked for me I wrote this eBook for you guys that would want to loose your weight within a short period of time. Sit back and enjoy the book.

CHAPTER ONE

What is intermittent fasting

Intermittent Fasting (IF) refers to dietary eating patterns that involves not eating or severely restricting calories for a prolonged period of time. There are many different subgroups of intermittent fasting each with individual variation in the duration of the fast; some for hours, others for day(s). This has become an extremely popular topic in the science community due to all of the potential benefits on fitness and health that are being discovered.

Fasting, or periods of voluntary abstinence from food has been practiced throughout the world for ages. Intermittent fasting with the goal of improving health relatively new. Intermittent fasting involves restricting intake of food for a set period of time and does not include any changes to the actual foods you are eating. Currently, the most common IF protocols are a daily 16 hour fast and fasting for a whole day, one or two days per week. Intermittent fasting could be considered a natural eating pattern that humans are built to implement and it traces all the way back to our paleolithic hunter-gatherer ancestors. The current model of a planned program of intermittent fasting could potentially help improve many aspects of health from body composition to longevity and aging. Although IF goes against the norms of our culture and common daily routine, the science may be pointing to less meal fre□uency and more time fasting as the optimal alternative to the normal breakfast, lunch, and dinner model. Here are two common myths that pertain to intermittent fasting.

First scenario - You Must Eat 3 Meals Per Day: This "rule" that is common in Western society was not developed based on evidence for improved health, but was adopted as the common pattern for settlers and eventually became the norm. Not only is there a lack of scientific rationale in the 3 meal-a-day model, recent studies may be showing less meals and more fasting to be optimal for human health. One study showed that one meal a day with the same number of daily calories is better for weight loss and body composition than 3 meals per day. This finding is a basic concept that is extrapolated into intermittent fasting and those choosing to do IF may find it best to only eat 1-2 meals per day.

Second scenario - You Need Breakfast, It's the Most Important Meal of The Day: Many false claims about the absolute need for a daily breakfast have been made. The most common claims being "breakfast increases your metabolism" and "breakfast decreases food intake later in the day". These claims have been refuted and studied over a 16-week period with results showing that skipping breakfast did not decrease metabolism and it did not increase food intake at lunch and dinner. It is still possible to do intermittent fasting protocols while still eating breakfast, but some people find it easier to eat a late breakfast or skip it altogether and this common myth should not get in the way.

CHAPTER TWO

How to do intermittent fasting properly

Let face it to understand how intermittent fasting leads to fat loss, we first need to understand the difference between the fed state and the fasted state.

Your body is in the fed state when it is digesting and absorbing food. Typically, the fed state starts when you begin eating and lasts for three to five hours as your body digests and absorbs the food you just ate. When you are in the fed state, it's very hard for your body to burn fat because your insulin levels are high.

After that timespan, your body goes into what is known as the post–absorptive state, which is just a fancy way of saying that your body isn't processing a meal. The post–absorptive state lasts until 8 to 12 hours after your last meal, which is when you enter the fasted state. It is much easier for your body to burn fat in the fasted state because your insulin levels are low.

When you're in the fasted state your body can burn fat that has been inaccessible during the fed state.

Because we don't enter the fasted state until 12 hours after our last meal, it's rare that our bodies are in this fat burning state. This is one of the reasons why many people who start intermittent fasting will lose fat without changing what they eat, how much they eat, or how often they exercise. Fasting puts your body in a fat burning state that you rarely make it to during a normal eating schedule.

CHAPTER THREE

The benefit of intermittent fasting

Fat loss is great, but it isn't the only benefit of intermittent fasting.

1. Intermittent fasting makes your day simpler.

I'm big on behavior change, simplicity, and reducing stress. Intermittent fasting provides additional simplicity to my life that I really enjoy. When I wake up, I don't worry about breakfast. I just grab a glass of water and start my day.

I enjoy eating and I don't mind cooking, so eating three meals a day was never a hassle for me. However, intermittent fasting allows me to eat one less meal, which also means planning one less meal, cooking one less meal, and stressing about one less meal. It makes life a bit simpler and I like that.

2. Intermittent fasting helps you live longer.

Scientists have long known that restricting calories is a way of lengthening life. From a logical standpoint, this makes sense. When you're starving, your body finds ways to extend your life.

There's just one problem: who wants to starve themselves in the name of living longer?

I don't know about you, but I'm interested in enjoying a long life. Starving myself doesn't sound that appetizing.

The good news is that intermittent fasting activates many of the same mechanisms for extending life as calorie restriction. In other words, you get the benefits of a longer life without the hassle of starving.

Way back in 1945 it was discovered that intermittent fasting extended life in mice. (Here's the study.) More recently, this study found that alternate day intermittent fasting led to longer lifespans.

3. Intermittent fasting may reduce the risk of cancer.

This one is up for debate because there hasn't been a lot of research and experimentation done on the relationship between cancer and fasting. Early reports, however, look positive.

This study of 10 cancer patients suggests that the side effects of chemotherapy may be diminished by fasting before treatment. This finding is also supported by another study which used alternate day fasting with cancer patients and concluded that fasting before chemotherapy would result in better cure rates and fewer deaths.

Finally, this comprehensive analysis of many studies on fasting and disease has concluded that fasting appears to not only reduce the risk of cancer, but also cardiovascular disease.

4. Intermittent fasting is much easier than dieting.

The reason most diets fail isn't because we switch to the wrong foods, it's because we don't actually follow the diet over the long term. It's not a nutrition problem, it's a behavior change problem.

This is where intermittent fasting shines because it's remarkably easy to implement once you get over the idea that you need to eat all the time. For example, this study found that intermittent fasting was an effective strategy for weight loss in obese adults and concluded that "subjects ⬚uickly adapt" to an intermittent fasting routine.

CHAPTER FOUR

The eating rules (Eat-stop-eat)

The eat-Stop-Eat method involves a 24-hour fast, either once or twice per week.

This method was popularized by fitness expert Brad Pilon, and has been ⬚uite popular for a few years.

By fasting from dinner one day, to dinner the next, this amounts to a 24-hour fast.

For example, if you finish dinner on Monday at 7 pm, and don't eat until dinner the next day at 7 pm, then you've just done a full 24-hour fast.

You can also fast from breakfast to breakfast, or lunch to lunch. The end result is the same.

Water, coffee and other non-caloric beverages are allowed during the fast, but no solid food.

If you are doing this to lose weight, then it is very important that you eat normally during the eating periods. As in, eat the same amount of food as if you hadn't been fasting at all.

The problem with this method is that a full 24-hour fast can be fairly difficult for many people.

However, you don't need to go all-in right away, starting with 14-16 hours and then moving upwards from there is fine.

I've personally done this a few times. I found the first part of the fast very easy, but in the last few hours I did become ravenously hungry.

I needed to apply some serious self-discipline to finish the full 24-hours and often found myself giving up and eating dinner a bit earlier.

CHAPTER FIVE

The things we can eat

There are millions of people who need to lose wight, and lose it right now because of poor health, and many of these people are searching for the best way to do this. What many people do not realize is that they already know within themselves how and what they should be doing to lose weight fast. Just consider this: if you put apple juice in your car, would it work as well as gasoline? No, and it's something you wouldn't dream of doing. But by putting junk foods in our bodies, we are not giving our bodies what they need to operate on efficiently, and our health will suffer.

Your body is a complex machine that is capable of doing so much, but it needs to have the correct foods to be able to do that, so what you eat becomes very important. It is even more important if you want to or need to lose weight because of the foods you have been eating, or the lack of exercise you've had. But the good news is that you can in fact eat to lose weight fast.

However eating to lose weight doesn't mean that you can eat any thing and everything around you without having to pay the consequences. If you continually eat fast food with its high fat content and lack of nutrition, then you should expect to gain weight. If you want to eat to lose weight, then try to change your diet, a little at a time, or all at once if you can. Cut out the high fat, high salt, high sugar foods, and your body will thank you for it later. You see, fast food isn't just high in fat, it also contains lots of sodium, salt, and the desserts are high in sugar too. The human body does not need very much sodium each day, and it can get its sugar from fruit, a healthier choice.

The Food and Drug Administration have set guidelines on what we should be eating each and every day, as well as the foods we shouldn't be, and they now have better information on every packaged product about what they contain. Now, not many people read the list of contents, or see how much sodium or sugar there is in a product, and you will probably be shocked to see just how much you are consuming that your body doesn't need. Next time you are shopping, take a look at the contents of some of the foods you regularly buy, or look at the tins or prepackaged foods you have at home. There are a lot of additives in foods to preserve them, and to make them taste better, but they are not necessarily good for you.

Okay, so what should you be eating to lose that weight? Go back to the basics, eating fruits and vegetables, fresh if possible, and whole grain cereals. Include protein which comes from meat, poultry and fish, but try to eat the low fat protein, as this will help your cholesterol levels. Eat nuts, and foods low in saturated fats, low in trans fats and cholesterol, as well as foods low in salt and sugar. And don't panic. This gives you a lot of options for variety in your meals, and enjoying different foods is a good thing to do, if the foods are recognized as healthy foods.

By eating healthy foods, you will be providing your body what it needs to operate efficiently, and you will feel healthier because you will be healthier. Drink plenty of water each day, after all, your body is made up of a lot of water to begin with. Don't over eat. We all do this, especially during those special times during the year, like Thanksgiving, and Christmas when we stuff ourselves with way too much food, and wonder why we nod off afterward. Our bodies just have such a hard time coping with these huge amounts of food.

Try to reduce your portion size if you need to lose weight, once you are eating the healthy foods that is, and don't forget to exercise. Your body was made and expects you to move about frequently during the day, so make sure your does. Try taking a brisk walk after a big meal, and do not lie down, use up some of those excess calories.

CHAPTER SIX

How to speed up your result by exercising

During the time you are doing the intermittent fasting there are exercises you must do in combination with fitness is probably the best way in losing weight. Losing weight is a thing many people want to do but most of them don't know exactly how to do this. They take a excessive diet and loose weight that they will gain again as soon as they stop with the diet. A diet will give you some rapid results but in the long term it will not help you much.

The first thing you need to do when you want to loose weight is changing your eating pattern This is not the same as taking a diet, as changing your eating pattern is something you should do permanent. After this, you could start with doing exercises. The best way in doing this is going to the gym and ask for a personal coach. He will help you making your personal schedule and decrease the chance on injury. Doing exercises will help you build up muscles and the good thing about muscles is that they will burn body fat rapidly. However, this is not enough for drastically losing weight. A good combination is doing fitness aside the exercises. When you do this, you will build up muscles and give your muscles the chance to burn the fat doing these fitness. A good way in doing this could be cycling or running. Both are easy to do as you can do it when and where you want.

The hardest part in losing weight is keeping up with your new lifestyle. Don't fall back in your old eating pattern or stop doing exercises when you reached your goal. It is very important to keep doing what you are doing.

www.ingramcontent.com/pod-product-compliance
Lightning Source LLC
Chambersburg PA
CBHW051409280526
45784CB00007B/3157